EMBRACE YOUR EMPATHY
AND LOVE YOUR GIFT

Mel Collins

Positive Affirmations for Sensitive People

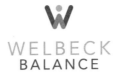

WELBECK
BALANCE

About the Author

MEL COLLINS is a qualified psychotherapeutic counsellor, spiritual life coach, healer, regression therapist – and highly sensitive person (HSP). She has run her own therapeutic and complementary healing practice for 18 years, specializing in working with HSPs and empaths.

Before becoming a counsellor, Mel worked in Her Majesty's Prison Service – including eight years as a prison governor. Being sensitive in a challenging prison setting provided her with unique insight into being an HSP and a frontline key worker.

Mel is a registered member of BAHA (British Alliance of Healing Associations) and a member of the Society of Authors. Her first book, *The Handbook for Highly Sensitive People*, has been translated into 11 languages. For further information please visit: **www.melcollins.co.uk**.

Published in 2022 by Welbeck Balance
An imprint of Trigger Ltd
Part of Welbeck Publishing Group.
Based in London and Sydney.
www.welbeckpublishing.com

Design and layout © Trigger Ltd 2022
Text © Mel Collins 2022

A CIP catalogue record for this book is available from the British Library

ISBN
Hardback – 978-1-80129-080-7

Typeset by Steve Williams Creative
Printed by RR Donnelley in Dongguan, China

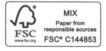

MIX
Paper from
responsible sources
FSC® C144853
FSC
www.fsc.org

Note/Disclaimer

Welbeck Balance encourages diversity and different viewpoints. However, all views,
thoughts, and opinions expressed in this book are the author's own and are not
necessarily representative of Welbeck Publishing Group as an organisation. All material
in this book is set out in good faith for general guidance; no liability can be accepted
for loss or expense incurred in following the information given. In particular, this
book is not intended to replace expert medical or psychiatric advice. It is intended
for informational purposes only and for your own personal use and guidance. It is not
intended to diagnose, treat or act as a substitute for professional medical advice.
The author is not a medical practitioner, and professional advice should be sought if
desired before embarking on any health-related programme.

www.welbeckpublishing.com

To sensitive people everywhere, and to those who help them feel less overwhelmed in this non-sensitive world.

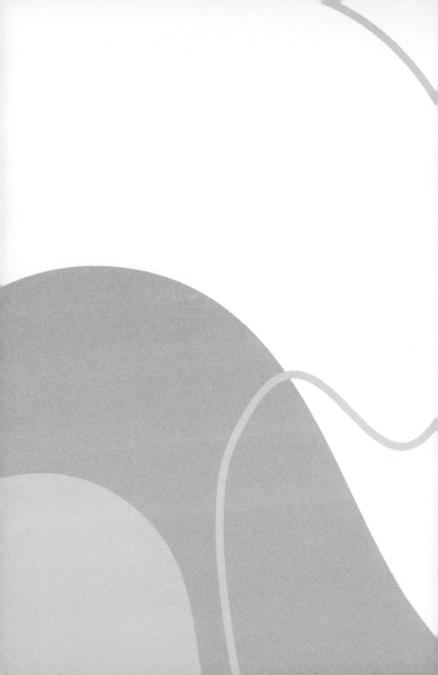

Introduction

I grew up thinking that there was something 'wrong' with me because I was so sensitive. I was also highly empathic, and I seemed to absorb other people's moods and feelings like a sponge. I could pick up on subtleties that others couldn't, and I seemed to process my emotions much more deeply than other people did.

Too much noise, being in crowds or not having any time or space to myself would leave me feeling frazzled and I would need to withdraw into nature in order to recharge.

I was often told that I was 'too sensitive for my own good', or that I should 'stop taking things to heart'. I was even told to 'toughen up', and in the end, that's what I did.

I internalized these messages as criticisms and came to believe that my sensitivity was not only a weakness but a massive flaw. I ended up wearing a strong, independent mask when I was around other people, and I locked parts of myself away for self-protection.

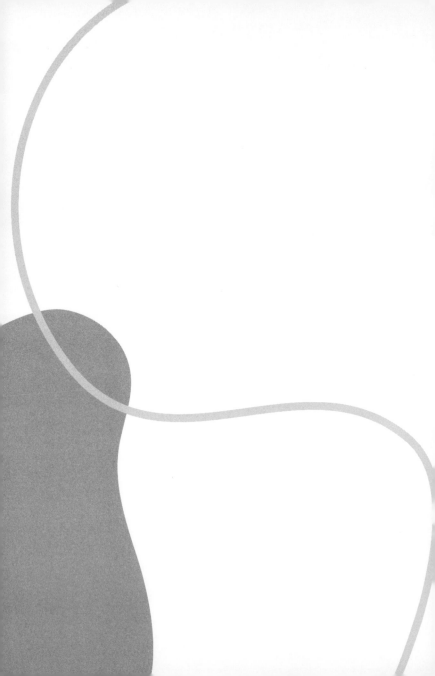

As a result, I became disconnected from my true self and felt lost inside for quite a few years.

When I was 31 years old, I got a part-time job in a prison, rehabilitating offenders. I know that sounds like a paradox for someone who is highly sensitive, but on reflection, I came to see that those messages to 'toughen up' simply got reflected into the environment where I worked. After a couple of years, I was promoted to a senior management role (a governor-grade position) and I jointly managed the Substance Misuse Services department and its strategic overview.

Thankfully, my intuition had guided me to train as a psychotherapeutic counsellor alongside my prison work. It was during the second year of this five-year training that I came across a book about 'high sensitivity'. I discovered that one in five people are born with this innate temperament trait, and every page of that book seemed to describe me perfectly. I finally realized that there was nothing actually 'wrong' with me. I was, in fact, just a Highly Sensitive Person (HSP).

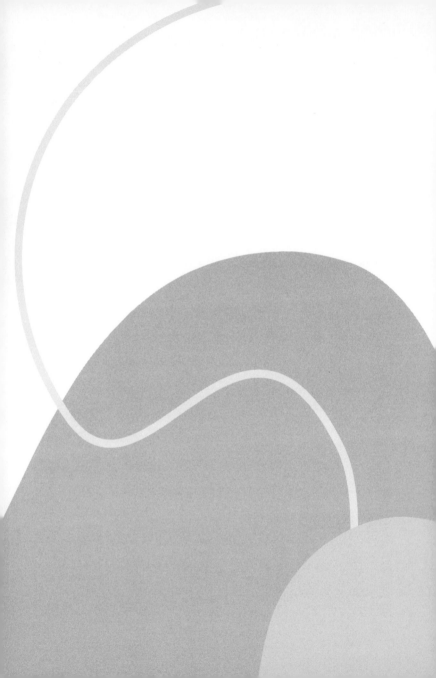

I began to understand my trait better and accept my sensitivity. I embraced it, along with its wonderful qualities. I was able to see it as a gift and a strength, and I felt more empowered. I decided to train in other healing modalities alongside my prison and counselling work and I have spent nearly two decades since working with HSP clients and carrying out my own research.

I also wrote *The Handbook for Highly Sensitive People* (Watkins Publishing, 2019), so that I could help many more HSPs to feel less frazzled and more empowered in this non-sensitive world.

Whether you consider yourself to be an HSP, an empath or just a sensitive person, I hope that by sharing the insights and positive affirmations in this book you will also feel more empowered. You may then see how your life starts to change for the better – just like mine did *once I embraced my sensitivity*.

Ten Signs that Indicate You Might Be an HSP

If you are wondering whether you are an HSP, the statements below can help you recognize whether you might have the trait. The more you answer yes, the more likely it is.

1. I am more reactive on an emotional level to events in my life or to the positive or negative emotions of others.
2. My feelings get hurt easily.
3. I'm sensitive to caffeine, strong smells, coarse fabrics and unnatural lighting.
4. I often feel overwhelmed by too much noise or in large groups of people and I find myself needing to withdraw to a quiet place.
5. I get affected by other people's moods and I can end up feeling drained, while others say they feel better after being with me.

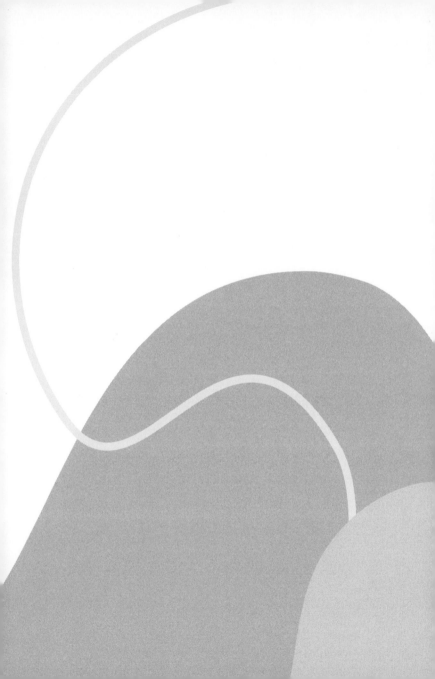

6. I find highly stimulating situations difficult and I don't perform as well if I'm being observed, taking a test or speaking in public.
7. I'm a natural giver and I struggle to implement boundaries.
8. I hate confrontation, and I deliberately avoid upsetting situations.
9. I tend to see the 'bigger picture'.
10. I am highly conscientious. I give great attention to detail or could be considered a perfectionist.

(Please note: the statements above are not meant to diagnose or exclude the diagnosis of any condition.)

If you need further clarity, the *Handbook* provides a comprehensive insight into the trait, the main indicators and a further self-help tick-list.

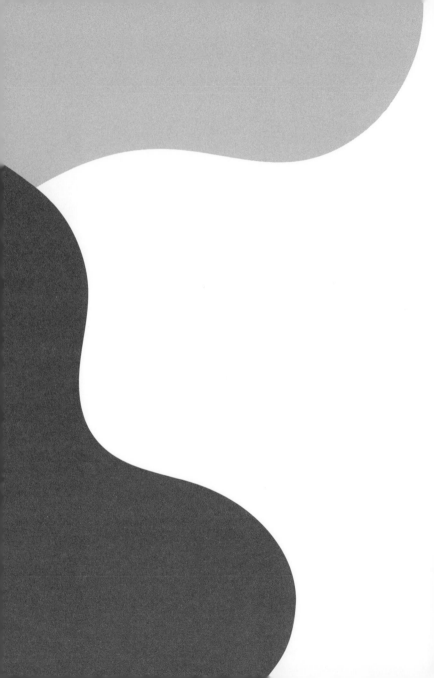

About This Book

This book contains a collection of personal insights from my own journey as an HSP and 100 associated positive affirmations that you can use – to not only understand and reframe some aspects of the trait, but to also help you embrace your sensitivity, consider it a gift and recognize the beautiful qualities associated with it.

The insights included not only show what I have learnt along the way, but they seem to reflect some universal truths and experiences within many HSPs, as I discovered through my research and therapy work.

My hope is that by sharing these insights, you will gain more awareness about the trait and start to feel more empowered as a result. Perhaps the affirmations will help you to uncover your own nuggets of wisdom, and reveal some insights of your own.

How to Use Affirmations

Affirmations are positive statements that are repeated often to challenge negative or unhelpful thoughts. With regular daily practice (for a minimum of 21 days), you can make lasting changes to the way you think and feel. Through repetition, the affirmations embed into the subconscious mind. Eventually, the negative beliefs fade, and the new positive ones become more believable and authentic.

You can either repeat an affirmation in your head or say it out loud. Many find that vocalizing the phrase gives power to the words. Some find that looking in a mirror while saying the affirmation makes a difference to how effective the affirmation feels, although this might seem a little strange at first! The added benefit of doing mirror work is that it can help to heal self-love issues.

Many people make affirmations a part of their daily routine – saying them out loud in front of a mirror first thing in the morning, before they start their day, and then again last thing at night before

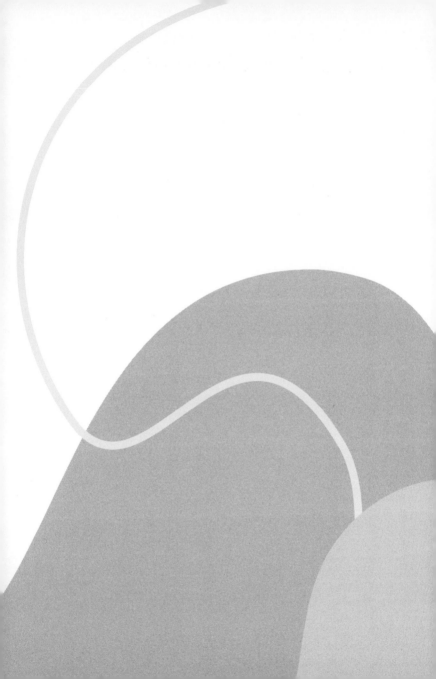

they go to sleep. It is recommended that you do this for at least five or ten minutes a day.

If your time is limited and you have a busy lifestyle, this structured approach may not work for you – and that's okay! Instead, you could write your favourite ones onto Post-it notes and place them around the house or next to your work computer. Then repeat them out loud or to yourself throughout the day when you come across them, or during breaks from work.

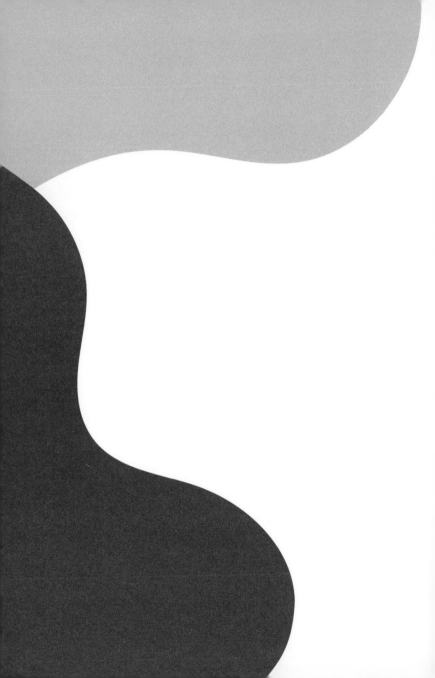

How to Use This Book

This book is designed so that you can dip in and find an affirmation that feels right for you in the moment.

You can either read from beginning to end and then choose two or three of your favourite affirmations to start working with, or just open the book on a random page and see which affirmation you have chosen intuitively.

If you want to go deeper, try reflecting or journaling on each insight so that you can uncover your own nuggets of wisdom. Notice any feelings, images or memories that come up for you and then take any new awareness from these insights into your everyday life. For example, giving yourself time and space to rest after a day of travelling rather than going straight out to explore or meet friends. This helps to reduce overstimulation in the sensory nervous system and prevents overarousal.

You can also use an affirmation as a mantra during meditation – it's a great way to help focus and still the mind.

*Once I embraced
my sensitivity,*

I realized it was my
greatest strength and not my
biggest weakness.

My sensitivity is my greatest strength.

*Once I embraced
my sensitivity,*

I realized that I wasn't 'flawed'
and that there was nothing
'wrong' with me.

*I love and
accept myself
exactly as I am.*

Once I embraced
my sensitivity,

I didn't feel so alone.
I learnt that 15 to 20
per cent of the population
are innately sensitive,
just like me.

That means there are
over 1.4 billion of us!

I am part of a worldwide community of highly sensitive people.

*Once I embraced
my sensitivity,*

I came to understand that I just process my emotions more deeply and for longer than others do.

(But that doesn't mean that we HSPs are better than anyone else!)

I am highly
reflective, and
I process my
emotions deeply.

*Once I embraced
my sensitivity,*

I chose not to let other people's
judgements, criticisms or
put-downs about being 'overly'
or 'hyper' sensitive affect my
self-esteem or eat away at
my self-worth.

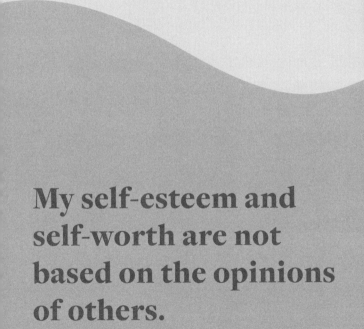

My self-esteem and self-worth are not based on the opinions of others.

*Once I embraced
my sensitivity,*

I started to heal deep-rooted
beliefs around my self-worth
and not being good enough.

I am good enough,
I am worthy, and I
deserve the best.

*Once I embraced
my sensitivity,*

I realized that I didn't
need to 'toughen up'.

(Maybe others could
soften instead?)

My gentleness
is a strength, and I
am no pushover.

*Once I embraced
my sensitivity,*

I came to see that not everyone
is able to pick up on subtleties
like I do, or notice small details.

I now regard my sensitivity as
one of my best skills.

I am able to pick up on subtleties – it's one of my superpowers!

*Once I embraced
my sensitivity,*

I realized that I wasn't shy
or fussy growing up, nor was
I a daydreamer – I was just
highly sensitive.

I am letting go of
the labels placed on
me as a child.

Once I embraced my sensitivity,

I no longer felt like an alien or the 'odd one out' in my family.

I accepted that I wasn't like the other members, and I stopped adapting myself to fit in.

I realized that being different wasn't a bad thing.

I am embracing
the diversity within
my family.

*Once I embraced
my sensitivity,*

I found a better balance between
being too much in the world and
being too much out of it.

Previously, if it was too much,
I would either shut down or
need to withdraw; if it was
too little, I ended up feeling
bored and uninspired.

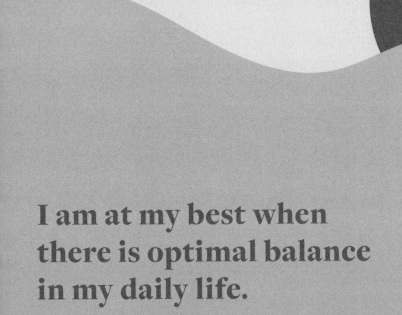

I am at my best when
there is optimal balance
in my daily life.

Once I embraced
my sensitivity,

I avoided the places that were too busy or too noisy, like shopping centres or crowds.

And if I couldn't avoid them, I limited the time I spent in these environments.

I enjoy spending time in places that are harmonious with my sensory nervous system.

Once I embraced
my sensitivity,

I scheduled rest breaks
into my diary.

Because being highly sensitive,
conscientious and a perfectionist
can be utterly exhausting when
it comes to work.

I am taking proper breaks at work because I perform better in the long run.

*Once I embraced
my sensitivity,*

I asked for a quiet office at work
because an open-plan set-up was
just too noisy and busy for me.

I am able to ask about making reasonable adjustments to support my wellbeing at work.

*Once I embraced
my sensitivity,*

I stopped ignoring my
body's messages of being
overstimulated.

As a result, I felt less frazzled
and overwhelmed.

I am listening to my body because it always lets me know when I need to rest and relax.

*Once I embraced
my sensitivity,*

I stopped thinking of myself
as boring because I couldn't
stay at parties all night like my
friends were able to do.

I socialize in a way that works for me.

*Once I embraced
my sensitivity,*

I loved it when people
who thought I was shy or aloof
when they first met me realized
that I was actually neither
of those things.

They came to understand that
for me, meeting strangers can
sometimes be overarousing for
my sensory nervous system.

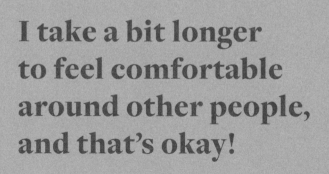

I take a bit longer
to feel comfortable
around other people,
and that's okay!

*Once I embraced
my sensitivity,*

I trusted my ability to
tune into other people
and pick up on what
they weren't saying.

I am able to tune into other people and know things without knowing how I know.

*Once I embraced
my sensitivity,*

I knew when people
weren't telling me the truth,
no matter how much they tried
to convince me otherwise.

My finely attuned senses
could pick up on their energy
and their lies.

I have finely attuned senses and a built-in lie detector – how amazing is that!

*Once I embraced
my sensitivity,*

I implemented boundaries.

Those people who tried to
put upon, control or manipulate
me didn't like them.

But I did. I only wish
I'd done it sooner.

I honour and respect myself by having healthy boundaries.

*Once I embraced
my sensitivity,*

I allowed myself to feel angry
instead of suppressing it. It didn't
mean I was being unkind.

Now I can express anger
by simply saying, 'I feel angry
about this,' or 'I felt angry when
you said or did that.'

I allow myself
to express my anger
in a healthy,
appropriate way.

*Once I embraced
my sensitivity,*

I owned ALL my feelings
instead of projecting the ones
I didn't like onto others.

I am owning my feelings, including the ones I dislike.

*Once I embraced
my sensitivity,*

I quit blaming others for
making me feel a certain way.

Now I understand that
no one can MAKE you feel
anything – they can only trigger
feelings that are already there.

I am becoming aware of my own triggers so I can respond, rather than react, if someone presses my buttons.

*Once I embraced
my sensitivity,*

I let go of old limiting beliefs
about being sensitive and
embraced new positive
ones instead.

I am creating new
positive beliefs
about sensitivity.

Once I embraced
my sensitivity,

I started to recognize
my own value.

I walked away from friendships
and relationships that didn't
respect my sensitivity.

It created the space
to find friends and lovers
who did.

I value myself, and
I attract others who
value me too.

*Once I embraced
my sensitivity,*

I learnt to receive as well as give.

Then I stopped attracting just
the 'takers' into my life.

I am in reciprocal relationships – where there is a healthy balance between giving and taking, listening and sharing.

*Once I embraced
my sensitivity,*

I walked away from people
who deliberately created
drama in my life.

I am choosing to walk away from toxic or unhealthy situations or relationships.

*Once I embraced
my sensitivity,*

I stopped taking on everyone's
problems as if they were mine
to fix.

I am not responsible for fixing other people's problems.

Once I embraced
my sensitivity,

I started to trust my intuition.

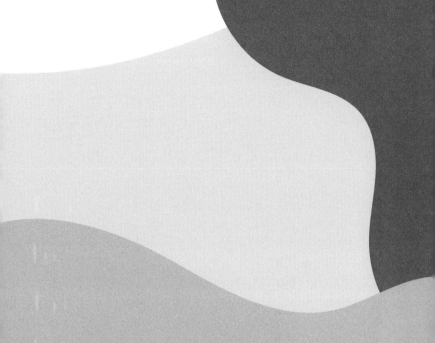

I (am learning to)
trust my intuition.

Once I embraced my sensitivity,

I realized how connected I was to the moon and its different phases.

The new and full moons would sometimes keep me awake all night. It used to frustrate me; now it doesn't. I just let myself bask in her beautiful light.

I am deeply connected to the moon.

My body and emotions are attuned to its natural cycles.

Once I embraced my sensitivity,

I spent much more time by the sea.

Ahh ... bliss!

I am calm
and stress-free.

Vitamin 'sea'
is good for me!

*Once I embraced
my sensitivity,*

I found nature was my sanctuary.

I also discovered the joy of forest
bathing. Sometimes I would
even hug trees.

(When nobody was looking,
of course!)

I am at peace in nature –
it's my sanctuary.

***Once I embraced
my sensitivity,***

I treasured my natural
connection to animals,
because of their unconditional
love and sensitivity.

I am deeply connected to animals.

*Once I embraced
my sensitivity,*

I tapped into my artistic and
creative abilities and found my
own way to express them.

I am expressing myself and my deepest emotions through ...

(dance, writing, singing, art, music etc.)

*Once I embraced
my sensitivity,*

I began to really value my levels
of empathy and compassion.

I am highly empathic and deeply compassionate, and these are beautiful qualities to have.

*Once I embraced
my sensitivity,*

I started protecting my
own energy.

I stopped absorbing other
people's moods and emotions
like a sponge. Then, instead
of feeling weighed down and
saturated, I began to feel lighter
and more buoyant again.

I am protecting my energy every day by visualizing myself inside a bubble of golden light.

Once I embraced my sensitivity,

I understood why I would walk into an environment and pick up on bad vibes or negative atmospheres.

I am able to pick up
on energies, so being in
positive environments
are best for me.

*Once I embraced
my sensitivity,*

I started to cleanse and purify
my aura and chakras regularly.

I am cleansing and purifying my energy field on a regular basis.

*Once I embraced
my sensitivity,*

I started walking barefoot on grass, soil or sand for ten minutes every day.

I discovered it was a good way of grounding myself.

I am grounded and 'earthed' when I am walking barefoot outside.

*Once I embraced
my sensitivity,*

I realized I was eating way too much chocolate – mainly for emotional comfort.

I've since cut down, but haven't given it up completely because I love it so much!

I am overcoming my comfort eating and finding healthier ways to meet my emotional needs.

*Once I embraced
my sensitivity,*

I cleaned up my diet and cut
out a lot of junk food.

I am honouring my body by eating nutritious food and drinking more water.

*Once I embraced
my sensitivity,*

I realized that my physical,
emotional, mental and
spiritual health were all
equally as important.

And all of them needed
to be kept in balance for
inner harmony.

I am healthy and vibrant. My physical, mental, emotional and spiritual health are all in balance.

Once I embraced
my sensitivity,

I learnt that making my own
needs a priority wasn't selfish
but self-loving.

When I discovered this,
I was able to help more
people, not less.

I am making my own needs a priority – because I can't give from an empty vessel.

*Once I embraced
my sensitivity,*

I stopped trying to fix or
rescue others.

I learnt it was a subconscious
way of trying to get my own
needs met.

*I am letting go
of the need to fix or
rescue others.*

*Once I embraced
my sensitivity,*

I stopped trying to change other people and changed the way I responded to them instead.

I am not able to change other people; I can only change the way I respond to them.

Once I embraced my sensitivity,

I stopped wearing a false mask around people in order to be more like them.

I don't need to be anyone else but me.

Authenticity is the key.

*Once I embraced
my sensitivity,*

I stopped being a people
pleaser ...

that one took a while!

I am learning how to be more assertive – because my wants, needs and happiness are just as important as other people's.

*Once I embraced
my sensitivity,*

I learnt to say NO without feeling guilty.

And when the 'ought to's or 'should's tried to creep back in, I would remind myself that these stem from other people's expectations.

I am able to say
NO and know it's
the right decision
for me.

Once I embraced
my sensitivity,

I started saying YES to things
that I really wanted to do.

I am saying YES
to things I really
want to do.

*Once I embraced
my sensitivity,*

I stopped trying to control
everything and went with the
flow instead.

I am going with the flow.

*Once I embraced
my sensitivity,*

I realized I was never going
to be perfect, so I stopped
trying to be!

I am perfectly imperfect!

*Once I embraced
my sensitivity,*
I listened to the wounded child
within me, and found ways to
nurture and heal her.

I lovingly parent and nurture my own inner child.

*Once I embraced
my sensitivity,*

I stopped going over the past
and worrying about the future
and started living in the present.

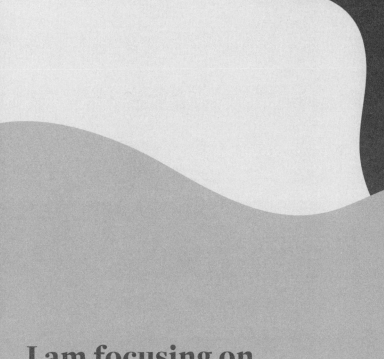

I am focusing on
being present and
living in the moment.

*Once I embraced
my sensitivity,*

I explored my fears and anxieties
consciously, so they didn't rule
my choices and decisions.

I am more than
my fears.

(But I can also ask
for help and support
to explore and
manage them if
I need to.)

*Once I embraced
my sensitivity,*

I realized that I had to stop
judging myself for mistakes I had
made along the way.

I am learning to
be more forgiving
toward myself.

*Once I embraced
my sensitivity,*

I stripped away the layers of hurt
and emotional pain that had
weighed me down.

I found inner freedom and
felt so much lighter.

*I am letting go of things
that weigh me down.*

*I am feeling lighter
every day.*

Once I embraced my sensitivity,

I learnt how to surf the waves when things got rough, rather than drown in them.

After all, waves reach a peak, and they always subside.

I am surfing the waves knowing that 'this too shall pass'.

Once I embraced my sensitivity,

I realized that I didn't have to 'prove' myself to anyone.

I have nothing to prove.

*Once I embraced
my sensitivity,*

I realized that there was
strength in vulnerability.

I allow myself to be
vulnerable with those
who can listen and
support me.

*Once I embraced
my sensitivity,*

I didn't care that I was teased
about crying during sad movies.

I am comfortable
with expressing
my emotions
and feelings.

*Once I embraced
my sensitivity,*

I was no longer triggered by people who told me to 'stop being so sensitive' – because I learnt that I can't stop something that is innate and natural.

Instead, I would ask them if they could stop having blue eyes – then they understood!

I am able to tell people to research what it means to be highly sensitive if they want to understand it or me better.

*Once I embraced
my sensitivity,*

I realized that those who
couldn't handle my emotions
were usually not in touch
with their own.

*I am more discerning
about who I can share my
emotions with.*

*Once I embraced
my sensitivity,*

I realized that I needn't feel
ashamed for being 'too much'
for some people.

I am never 'too much' for the right people.

Once I embraced
my sensitivity,

I realized that those people who triggered the strongest reactions in me were just mirroring something that needed to be healed within myself.

I am committed to my personal growth.

I consciously explore my triggers and reactions so that I can heal them.

***Once I embraced
my sensitivity,***

I explored my shadow and
welcomed back the parts of
me that had been deemed
unacceptable by others or
felt shamed.

Something amazing happens
when you shine the light on
them ... these parts stop acting
out in unconscious ways.

And then I began to feel
whole again.

I accept myself fully.

I understand that light and darkness exist within us all.

*Once I embraced
my sensitivity,*

I befriended my 'Inner Critic' ...
but it took a long time.

(And we still have the
occasional fallout!)

My Inner Critic
becomes more and
more quiet as I
question the validity
of its comments.

I am learning to
speak more kindly
to myself.

Once I embraced my sensitivity,

I found my power and stopped feeling like a victim.

I am taking back my power.

Once I embraced my sensitivity,

I supported the 'underdogs' even more because of my strong sense of social justice.

*I am an advocate
of social justice, fairness
and equality.*

*Once I embraced
my sensitivity,*

I stopped comparing
myself to others.

I am me, and
you are you.

There is no need to
compare the two.

*Once I embraced
my sensitivity,*

I challenged those who called
HSPs 'snowflakes' or other
derogatory names.

I told them that sensitive people
are some of the strongest
they'll ever meet, because it
takes great strength to remain
compassionate when people are
being unkind or cruel.

I am able to feel compassion because I can see behind people's behaviours.

I also know that love and kindness are far more powerful than fear and negativity.

*Once I embraced
my sensitivity,*

I formed deep roots so that
other people or difficult
experiences wouldn't knock
me down again.

I am building
solid foundations
within myself.

Once I embraced my sensitivity,

I developed a stronger sense of self.

I understand my trait, and this gives me a stronger sense of self.

Once I embraced
my sensitivity,

I unlocked the gates
around my heart.

My fear of being badly hurt
again had become a form of
self-imprisonment and had kept
me in solitary confinement.

I am more discerning when it comes to potential relationships. I am trusting my gut instincts, and I am no longer ignoring any red flags or inner alarm bells.

*Once I embraced
my sensitivity,*

I realized that overthinking was part of the sensitivity trait. But I also realized that there were different ways to silence my mind and stop the carousel of thoughts going around my head.

I am able to quiet my mind through meditation or mindfulness.

*Once I embraced
my sensitivity,*

I would focus on my breathing
when I was overwhelmed or
during difficult times because
I was a 'holder'.

Now I focus on 'letting go' with
my breath, by inhaling and
exhaling deeply. It's one of the
easiest and best strategies to
reduce overarousal.

I am breathing in peace (on the inhale)

and breathing out stress (on the exhale).

*Once I embraced
my sensitivity,*

I realized I wasn't the only one
who dreaded public speaking –
many sensitive people do.

But now I feel the fear and
do it anyway.

I am practising my speeches so that I am more confident of doing them in public.

Once I embraced my sensitivity,

I discovered that most of us HSPs can't watch horror movies or violent films.

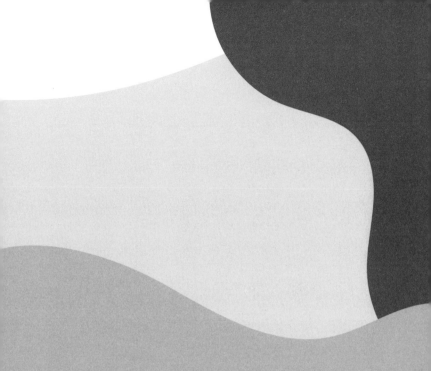

I am a lover of
feel-good movies.

Once I embraced my sensitivity,

I understood why I felt so much pain and sadness about the destruction taking place on our planet.

I am taking positive action and making changes to the way I live to help protect the planet.

Once I embraced

my sensitivity,

I discovered that having a rich
and complex inner life was
natural for HSPs.

I love my inner world –
it's a fascinating place
and I enjoy spending
time there!

*Once I embraced
my sensitivity,*

I realized that many highly
sensitive people have vivid,
prophetic or lucid dreams
like I do.

*I am still processing
my emotions and
receiving guidance even
in my dreams.*

Once I embraced my sensitivity,

I stopped questioning why complete strangers would pour their hearts out to me.

I am a good listener and people feel safe opening up to me.

***Once I embraced
my sensitivity,***

I developed my natural
healing and psychic abilities
so I could be of help and
service to others.

I am using my gifts and abilities to help others.

Once I embraced my sensitivity,

I started to thrive rather than just survive in this non-sensitive world.

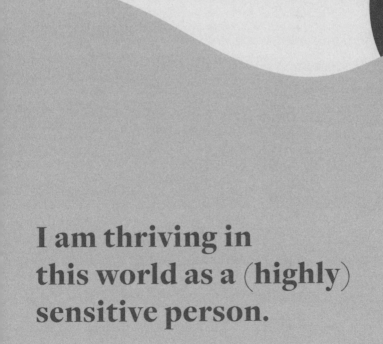

I am thriving in
this world as a (highly)
sensitive person.

Once I embraced
my sensitivity,

I began to live from my heart
again and not just my head.

I am living my life in a heart-centred and mindful way.

Once I embraced
my sensitivity,

I forgave myself for all the times
and ways I had dishonoured it.

I forgive myself for not honouring my sensitivity in the past.

*Once I embraced
my sensitivity,*

I decided to teach others
how to embrace their own.

I am embracing my sensitivity and helping others to embrace theirs too.

*Once I embraced
my sensitivity,*

I discovered a mind-body-spirit connection.

And I started to take more notice of what my higher self was trying to tell me through my body and feelings – instead of ignoring their messages.

I am learning to tune in and listen to my higher self – the wise, all-knowing part of me.

Once I embraced my sensitivity,

I started to meditate regularly. It enabled me to hear the whispers of my soul and its innate wisdom much more easily.

I am able to access higher guidance through meditation.

*Once I embraced
my sensitivity,*

I came to see that being called
a 'sensitive soul' as a child was,
in fact, a compliment and
not a criticism.

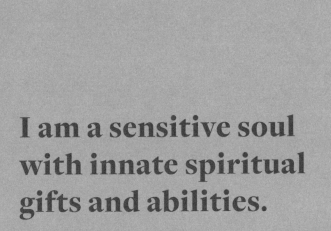

I am a sensitive soul
with innate spiritual
gifts and abilities.

Once I embraced my sensitivity,

That deep feeling of 'homesickness' (like I didn't belong here on this planet) got easier to live with.

I am a soul with
a divine purpose
to fulfil.

Once I embraced
my sensitivity,

I started to focus on my passions, and then my dreams started to become a reality.

I am following my passions and making my dreams come true.

*Once I embraced
my sensitivity,*

I searched for the gifts and
lessons in my challenges.

I realized that obstacles
were there to help me grow
and evolve, both personally
and spiritually.

I am finding the gifts and lessons in my challenges.

*Once I embraced
my sensitivity,*

I kept working on the three Ss:

Self-acceptance, Self-care
and Self-love.

Because I understood I was
a work-in-progress.

I am learning to love
and accept myself,
and make self-care
a priority.

Once I embraced my sensitivity,

I realized that it didn't matter if people understood my sensitivity – it only mattered that I did.

I understand my sensitivity and it's okay if others don't.

*Once I embraced
my sensitivity,*

I realized that many countries
and cultures truly value
sensitive people.

(But the Western world still
has a lot of catching up to do!)

I am thankful that sensitivity is truly valued in many cultures and countries.

*Once I embraced
my sensitivity,*

I started to align with
my true self.

Now I live more authentically.

I am aligning
with my true self
and living a more
authentic life.

Once I embraced
my sensitivity,

I deepened my relationship
with a higher power/God, and I
strengthened my connection to
the spiritual beings who guide
and protect me.

I am a child of God, and my spirit guides and angels are always with me.

*Once I embraced
my sensitivity,*

I grieved deeply for the people
I loved who had passed to spirit.
The ones who truly 'got' me.

But I also knew they were still
around – because I could sense
and feel them there.

Now they help me from the 'other
side'. What a blessing that is.

I am supported and guided by my loved ones in the spirit world.

Once I embraced my sensitivity,

I recognized it as an expression of love.

My sensitivity is an expression of love.

*Once I embraced
my sensitivity,*

I loved the gift of sensitivity,
instead of seeing it as a
weakness or a flaw.

I feel blessed and grateful for the gift of sensitivity.

ABOUT US

Welbeck Balance publishes books dedicated to changing lives. Our mission is to deliver life-enhancing books to help improve your wellbeing so that you can live your life with greater clarity and meaning, wherever you are on life's journey. Our Trigger books are specifically devoted to opening up conversations about mental health and wellbeing.

Welbeck Balance and Trigger are part of the Welbeck Publishing Group – a globally recognized independent publisher based in London. Welbeck are renowned for our innovative ideas, production values and developing long-lasting content. Our books have been translated into over 30 languages in more than 60 countries around the world.

If you love books, then join the club and sign up to our newsletter for exclusive offers, extracts, author interviews and more information.

www.welbeckpublishing.com   www.triggerhub.org

🐦 welbeckpublish   🐦 Triggercalm
📷 welbeckpublish   📷 Triggercalm
f welbeckuk   f Triggercalm

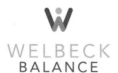

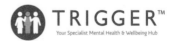